GLAUCOMA PREVENTION DIET COOKBOOK

Nutrition Strategies For Healthy Vision-Delicious Recipes For Eye Health -Empower Your Eyes With Smart Eating

DR. SHAYLA LEWIS

Table of Contents

DISCLAIMER

Write a brief complete Disclaimer for my diet cook book telling them that the author is not in any association with any company, business or individual and also this book is written by the authors knowledge and understanding

The information provided in this diet cookbook is based on the author's personal knowledge and understanding. The author is not affiliated with, endorsed by, or associated with any company, business, or individual. The recipes and dietary advice contained within this book are intended for informational purposes only. Readers should consult with a healthcare professional or a registered dietitian before making any significant changes to their diet or lifestyle. The author assumes no responsibility for any adverse effects that may result from the use or misuse of the information contained in this book.

CHAPTER ONE

Understanding Glaucoma: An Overview

Glaucoma is a collection of eye disorders that cause damage to the optic nerve, usually due to increasing pressure inside the eye. If not treated, this injury might lead to vision loss and blindness.

The problem frequently develops slowly and may not create apparent symptoms until later stages, therefore annual eye exams are essential for early detection.

What is glaucoma and what are the different types?

Glaucoma has various kinds, but the two most common are open-angle glaucoma and angle-closure glaucoma.

Open-angle glaucoma is the most prevalent type, characterized by a steady increase in intraocular pressure produced by the slow blockage of the eye's drainage canals. It grows gradually over time and may not show symptoms until severe damage has occurred.

Angle-closure glaucoma develops when the iris becomes too close to the drainage angle in the eye, resulting in an abrupt occlusion of the drainage canals. This causes a rapid increase in intraocular pressure, necessitating quick medical intervention to avoid vision loss.

Other less common kinds are normal-tension glaucoma, congenital glaucoma, and secondary glaucoma, which can develop as a result of other eye problems or other difficulties.

How does glaucoma affect vision?

Glaucoma initially affects peripheral vision, then progresses to central vision as the condition worsens. Increased intraocular pressure harms the optic nerve, which transmits visual information from the eye to the brain. As nerve fibers are destroyed, the visual field shrinks, resulting in blind spots. Without treatment, glaucoma can eventually cause blindness.

Early identification is crucial in the management of glaucoma since once eyesight is lost, it cannot be recovered. Regular eye exams, particularly for people over the age of 40 or those with a family history of glaucoma, can help diagnose the disease early on when treatment is most successful.

Medication, laser therapy, and surgical procedures are used as prevention techniques to lower intraocular pressure. Furthermore, lifestyle changes such as keeping a healthy weight, exercising regularly, and quitting smoking will help lower your chance of developing glaucoma.

The role of nutrition in managing glaucoma

Nutrition alone cannot prevent or cure glaucoma, but it can help manage the illness and reduce the risk of progression. Certain foods have been linked to improved eye health and decreased intraocular pressure. This includes:

Antioxidants include vitamins C and E, zinc, and selenium, which help protect the eyes from oxidative stress and free radical damage. Antioxidant-rich foods include fruits, vegetables, nuts, and seeds.

Omega-3 fatty acids, found in fatty fish such as salmon, mackerel, and trout, have anti-inflammatory qualities that may help lower intraocular pressure and enhance general eye health.

Vitamin A: Carrots, sweet potatoes, spinach, and kale contain vitamin A, which is essential for keeping good vision. It improves retinal function and may lower the risk of glaucoma progression.

Bilberry: This antioxidant-rich fruit is frequently recommended for its possible eye health advantages, which include increased blood flow to the optic nerve and lower intraocular pressure.

Green tea: High in antioxidants known as catechins, green tea may protect the eyes and lower the risk of glaucoma progression.

While integrating these nutrients into a healthy diet may be useful for those with glaucoma, it's critical to speak with a doctor before making any big dietary changes.

They can make tailored recommendations depending on individual health status and dietary requirements. Adherence to prescribed medication and regular eye exams are still important aspects of glaucoma care.

CHAPTER TWO

Understanding the fundamentals of nutrition is critical to maintaining general health, including eye health. Nutrition provides the body with the nutrients it requires for tissue growth, repair, and maintenance, as well as internal activities. Proper nutrition is important for preventing glaucoma, a disorder characterized by elevated pressure in the eye that causes optic nerve damage.

Antioxidants such as vitamins C and E, beta-carotene, lutein, zeaxanthin, and omega-3 fatty acids are important nutrients for eye health and may help prevent or reduce the advancement of glaucoma. These nutrients serve to protect the eyes from oxidative stress, inflammation, and free radical damage.

A balanced diet is critical for general health and well-being, including eye health. It entails eating a range of meals from different food categories to ensure that the body gets all of the nutrients it requires in the proper proportions. A balanced diet usually includes:

Fruits and vegetables include high levels of vitamins, minerals, antioxidants, and dietary fiber. To maximize nutrient intake, aim to eat a colorful array of fruits and vegetables.

Whole Grains: Whole grains provide complex carbs, fiber, vitamins, and minerals. Choose whole grains such as brown rice, quinoa, whole wheat bread, and oats over refined grains.

Lean Protein: Protein is required for tissue repair and muscular building. Choose lean protein sources such as chicken, fish, tofu, beans, lentils, and nuts.

Healthy Fats: Omega-3 fatty acids found in fatty fish such as salmon, walnuts, flaxseeds, and chia seeds are good for your eyes and may help lower your risk of glaucoma.

Dairy products and dairy alternatives contain calcium, vitamin D, and other elements that are beneficial to bone health. Choose low-fat or nonfat dairy products or dairy alternatives such as fortified plant-based milk.

Limit Added Sugars and Sodium: Too much sugar and sodium in the diet can lead to a variety of health issues, including diabetes and high blood pressure, both of which are risk factors for glaucoma.

The Effect of Diet on Overall Health:
Diet is important for general health, and what you eat can influence many elements of your well-being, including your chance of acquiring chronic diseases such as diabetes, heart disease, and even eye conditions like

glaucoma. A bad diet high in processed foods, unhealthy fats, and added sweets can lead to inflammation, oxidative stress, and other risk factors for glaucoma.

A nutrient-dense diet, on the other hand, can give the body the critical nutrients it requires to maintain good health and possibly minimize the risk of getting glaucoma or slowing its progression.

Introducing Low-Carb, Antioxidant-Rich, and Anti-Inflammatory Foods:

Low-carb, antioxidant-rich, and anti-inflammatory meals can help prevent glaucoma.

Low-Carb Foods: While there is no clear evidence relating low-carb diets to glaucoma prevention, limiting refined carbohydrate and sugar consumption may help control underlying illnesses such as diabetes and obesity, both of which are risk factors for glaucoma.

Antioxidant-Rich Foods: Antioxidants help protect cells from free radical damage, including those in the eyes. Antioxidants like vitamin C (found in citrus fruits, strawberries, and bell peppers), vitamin E (found in nuts, seeds, and leafy greens), and carotenoids like lutein and zeaxanthin (found in spinach, kale, and other leafy greens) can help with eye health and may lower the risk of glaucoma.

Anti-inflammatory Foods: Chronic inflammation may contribute to the development and progression of glaucoma. Consuming anti-inflammatory foods such as fatty fish high in omega-3 fatty acids, turmeric, ginger, green tea, and colorful fruits and vegetables can help reduce inflammation and improve overall health, including vision.

To summarise, eating a well-balanced diet rich in nutrient-dense foods, such as low-carbohydrate alternatives, antioxidant-rich meals, and anti-inflammatory foods, can help prevent or manage glaucoma and improve general eye health. This Glaucoma Prevention Diet Cookbook seeks to provide delicious and nutritious dishes that follow these concepts to assist individuals in maintaining healthy vision and lowering their chance of acquiring eye disorders such as glaucoma.

Navigating Glaucoma and Related Conditions.

Glaucoma, also known as the "silent thief of sight," is a set of eye disorders that damage the optic nerve, usually as a result of increased pressure within the eye. If not addressed, the illness can develop into irreversible vision loss and blindness.

Understanding the various forms, symptoms, and treatment choices for glaucoma and related disorders is essential for navigating their intricacies.

Common Symptoms and Signs of Glaucoma

Glaucoma usually develops gradually and without obvious symptoms in the early stages. However, when the illness advances, people may encounter:

Gradual Loss of Peripheral Vision: This is frequently the first indication of glaucoma. As the optic nerve is injured, peripheral (side) vision begins to deteriorate.

hazy Vision: People may suffer from hazy vision or see halos surrounding lights.

Eye discomfort or Headaches: Some glaucoma patients may have mild to moderate eye discomfort or headaches, especially during acute episodes of high intraocular pressure.

Redness in the eye, especially if it is accompanied by pain or blurred vision, may indicate acute angle-closure glaucoma, which is a medical emergency.

5. Nausea and vomiting: These symptoms may coexist with acute angle-closure glaucoma due to the abrupt increase in ocular pressure.

Early identification of glaucoma is critical to preventing vision loss. Regular eye exams, including comprehensive dilated eye exams, are critical for diagnosing glaucoma before it causes major vision loss.

Understanding Neuropathy's Relationship with Diabetes

Neuropathy is a type of nerve injury that causes pain, numbness, and weakness, most commonly in the hands and feet. Diabetes is a prevalent cause of neuropathy because elevated blood sugar levels damage nerve fibers throughout the body.

The link between neuropathy and diabetes is complex. Prolonged periods of high blood sugar can harm the tiny blood vessels that feed nerves with oxygen and nutrients, resulting in nerve damage. This damage can lead to numerous kinds of neuropathy, including:

Peripheral Neuropathy is the most frequent type of neuropathy among diabetics. It usually affects the feet and legs first, giving symptoms like numbness, tingling, burning, and muscle weakness.

Autonomic Neuropathy: This type of neuropathy affects the autonomic nerve system, which regulates involuntary body activities like heart rate, digestion, and urination. Symptoms can include dizziness, fainting, nausea, vomiting, diarrhea, constipation, sexual dysfunction, and sweating issues.

Proximal neuropathy, also called diabetic amyotrophy, affects the thighs, hips, buttocks, and legs. Symptoms may include extreme discomfort, muscle weakness, and difficulty walking.

Managing neuropathy in diabetes entails keeping blood sugar levels under tight control while also addressing symptoms with medication, lifestyle changes, and alternative therapies.

Strategies to Manage Nerve Pain and Symptoms

Managing nerve pain and neuropathy symptoms, particularly those associated with glaucoma and diabetes necessitates a multifaceted approach that tackles both the underlying cause and the symptoms itself.

CHAPTER THREE

Here are some ways to control nerve pain and symptoms

Medications: Anticonvulsants, antidepressants, and pain relievers may help relieve nerve discomfort caused by neuropathy. However, it is critical to collaborate closely with a healthcare expert to determine the most effective and safe treatment plan.

Lifestyle changes, such as regular exercise, maintaining a healthy weight, stopping smoking, and avoiding excessive alcohol use, can all assist in enhancing nerve health and lessen neuropathy symptoms.

Dietary Changes: A nutritious diet high in fruits, vegetables, whole grains, lean protein, and healthy fats helps improve nerve health and general well-being. According to some studies, certain dietary supplements, such as alpha-lipoic acid and omega-3 fatty acids, may help alleviate neuropathic pain.

Alternative Therapies: Acupuncture, massage therapy, yoga, and biofeedback may help people with neuropathy relieve pain and enhance their overall quality of life.

Physical therapy helps improve strength, flexibility, and balance, lowering the risk of neuropathy-related falls and accidents.

Individuals with neuropathy must work together with their healthcare provider to build a personalized treatment plan that matches their specific requirements and goals.

The importance of holistic approaches to health

Holistic approaches to health emphasize the interconnectedness of the mind, body, and spirit, acknowledging that all areas of a person's life contribute to their overall well-being. When it comes to managing chronic illnesses like glaucoma, diabetes, and neuropathy, a holistic approach might be very helpful.

Holistic health treats the whole person, not just the symptoms of an illness. This may involve:

Nutrition: A good diet is critical for maintaining overall health and controlling chronic diseases. A nutrient-dense diet helps improve eye health, manage blood sugar levels, and promote neuron activity.

Physical Activity: Regular exercise not only helps to maintain a healthy weight and blood sugar levels, but it also improves circulation, decreases inflammation, and promotes nerve health.

Stress Management: Chronic stress can aggravate the symptoms of glaucoma, diabetes, and neuropathy. Meditation, deep breathing exercises, yoga, and tai chi are all stress-reduction strategies that can help you relax and feel better overall.

Sleep Hygiene: Adequate sleep is critical for overall health and well-being. Poor sleep quality or insufficient sleep can exacerbate symptoms of chronic illnesses and decrease overall functioning.

Mind-Body Practices: Mindfulness, meditation, and guided imagery can help people manage pain, and stress, and enhance their general well-being.

Individuals who embrace holistic approaches to health can empower themselves to actively manage their diseases and improve their overall well-being. This may entail making lifestyle changes, getting medical advice, and researching complementary therapies that address the physical, emotional, and spiritual components of health.

The Importance of Diet in Glaucoma Prevention

How nutrition affects eye health

The importance of antioxidants and their sources

Impact of inflammation on glaucoma progression

Adding low-carb meals to your diet.

The role of diet in glaucoma prevention:

Diet plays an important impact in general health, including eye health. Dietary choices can have a substantial impact on the risk of glaucoma and its progression. According to research, some nutrients and dietary patterns may minimize the likelihood of getting glaucoma or limit its progression in people who have already been diagnosed.

A diet high in antioxidants, vitamins, minerals, and healthy fats can improve optic nerve function and lower intraocular pressure, which is a major risk factor for glaucoma. Additionally, keeping a healthy weight through balanced nutrition might reduce the chance of acquiring illnesses such as diabetes and hypertension, both of which have been related to an increased risk of glaucoma.

A diet rich in whole foods and nutrient-dense nutrients can promote cardiovascular health and reduce oxidative stress, potentially lowering the incidence of glaucoma-related visual loss.

The proverb "you are what you eat" applies to eye health as well. Our diets contain critical nutrients that promote the function and structure of the eyes. Vitamins A, C, and E, omega-3 fatty acids, zinc, and antioxidants are essential for preserving eye health and preventing glaucoma.

For example, vitamin A is required for the formation of rhodopsin, a pigment in the retina that aids in low-light vision. Vitamin C promotes the health of the blood vessels in the eyes, whereas vitamin E protects cells from oxidative damage. Omega-3 fatty acids, present in fatty fish such as salmon and mackerel, are essential for retinal development and function.

By integrating a range of nutrient-dense foods into your diet, you can promote good eye health and lower your risk of glaucoma.

Antioxidants are crucial in protecting the eyes from oxidative stress, which can contribute to the development and progression of glaucoma. Oxidative stress occurs when the body's free radicals and antioxidants are out of equilibrium, causing cell and tissue damage, including that of the eyes.

Fruits, vegetables, nuts, seeds, and certain seasonings contain antioxidants. Vitamin C-rich foods, such as oranges, strawberries, and bell peppers, are powerful antioxidants that can protect the eyes from harm. Similarly, foods high in vitamin E, such as almonds, sunflower seeds, and spinach, can neutralize free radicals and lessen oxidative stress.

Other antioxidant-rich meals include kale and collard greens, which contain lutein and zeaxanthin, antioxidants that are especially good for your eyes

CHAPTER FOUR
The Impact of Inflammation on Glaucoma Progression

Chronic inflammation has been linked to the etiology of several illnesses, including glaucoma. Inflammation can damage the optic nerve and hasten the progression of the disease, resulting in vision loss over time.

Certain dietary variables can cause or lessen inflammation in the body. Diets strong in processed foods, refined carbs, and unhealthy fats have been related to increased inflammation, whereas diets rich in whole foods, fruits, vegetables, and omega-3 fatty acids have anti-inflammatory properties.

Adopting an anti-inflammatory diet can help reduce the impact of inflammation on glaucoma progression. This entails consuming fewer inflammatory items such as sugary snacks, processed meats, and fried foods while emphasizing complete, nutrient-dense foods that promote general health and well-being.

Low-carb diets can help people control their blood sugar levels and lower their risk of illnesses like diabetes, which is a major risk factor for glaucoma. By limiting your intake of refined carbohydrates and sweets, you can help stabilize blood glucose levels and improve overall metabolic health.

Incorporating low-carb dishes into your diet does not imply compromising flavor or diversity. Salads, stir-fries, grilled meats, and vegetables, as well as hearty soups and stews, are all wonderful and nutritious options. Focusing on protein-rich foods, healthy fats, and non-starchy veggies will help you feel full and content while also supporting your eye health and lowering your risk of glaucoma.

Furthermore, replacing high-carb items with low-carb equivalents allows you to enjoy your favorite foods without jeopardizing your health goals. Using cauliflower rice instead of white rice, lettuce wraps instead of tortillas, or zucchini noodles instead of pasta, for example, can help you cut carbs while adding nutrition and flavor to your meals.

Overall, adding low-carb meals into your diet can be a useful and successful method for maintaining good eye health and lowering your risk of glaucoma.

Getting Started: Essential Kitchen Tools and Ingredients

Must-have kitchen equipment for easy cooking:

A well-equipped kitchen will help you prepare glaucoma-friendly meals in an efficient and pleasurable manner. Here are some important gadgets to consider:

Vegetable Spiralizer: This equipment lets you make noodle-like shapes out of veggies including zucchini, carrots, and sweet potatoes. It's ideal for adding diversity to your meals while increasing your consumption of healthful vegetables.

Blender or Food Processor: A high-quality blender or food processor is required for making smoothies, soups, and sauces. These tools can help you add a variety of nutrient-dense foods to your diet, including leafy greens, fruits, and nuts.

Slow Cooker or Instant Pot: These flexible machines are perfect for creating nutritious meals with little effort. You can use them to cook grains, legumes, and lean proteins like chicken or fish, making it easy to incorporate these items into your glaucoma-prevention diet.

Non-stick Cookware: Purchasing non-stick pots and pans can make cooking easier while reducing the need for additional fats and oils. Look for cookware with robust, scratch-resistant coatings that are simple to clean.

Kitchen Scale: Measuring ingredients correctly is essential for following recipes and controlling portion proportions. A digital kitchen scale can help you keep track of the things you eat, such as grains, nuts, and seeds, which are essential components of a glaucoma-friendly diet.

Important elements for glaucoma-friendly meals:

When it comes to preventing glaucoma with diet, nutrient-dense foods are essential. Here are some crucial components to include in your meals:

Leafy Greens: Dark leafy greens such as spinach, kale, and collard greens include antioxidants such as lutein and zeaxanthin, which have been demonstrated to improve eye health and lower the risk of glaucoma.

Omega-3-rich foods, such as salmon, mackerel, flaxseeds, and walnuts, can help prevent glaucoma by lowering inflammation and boosting blood flow to the eyes.

Colourful fruits and vegetables, such as oranges, carrots, bell peppers, and berries, are high in vitamins, minerals, and antioxidants, which promote overall eye health and lower the chance of glaucoma damage.

Whole Grains: Choose whole grains like quinoa, brown rice, oats, and barley, which include fiber, vitamins, and minerals that promote healthy blood flow and lower the risk of eye problems such as glaucoma.

Lean Proteins: Incorporate lean protein sources into your meals, such as poultry, tofu, beans, and lentils, to promote muscle strength and keep blood sugar levels steady, which is essential for eye health.

Tips for Shopping and Meal Planning:

Efficient grocery shopping and meal preparation can help you keep organized while also ensuring that you have the necessary ingredients to produce glaucoma-friendly meals. Here are some suggestions to consider:

Make a List: Before you go grocery shopping, make a list of the ingredients you'll need for the coming week. To make your shopping trip more efficient, organize your list by food group.

Shop the Perimeter: Look around the supermarket store for fresh produce, lean proteins, and healthful grains. Limit your time in the center aisles, which are typically filled with processed and packaged items.

When fresh fruits and vegetables are unavailable, choose frozen or canned alternatives. These ingredients are frequently equally as nutritious and more convenient to keep on hand for quick and easy meal preparation.

Batch Cooking: Consider cooking big amounts of grains, beans, and proteins at the start of the week to use in numerous meals. This saves time and ensures that you have nutritious options available throughout the week.

Experiment with New Recipes: To make mealtime more exciting, try new recipes and experiment with different ingredients and flavor combinations. Look for glaucoma-friendly recipes online or in cookbooks to make your meals interesting and diverse.

How to Make Cooking Fun and Stress-Free:

Cooking can be a relaxing and joyful activity, especially when tackled with the proper attitude. Here are some ideas to make cooking stress-free:

Create a Relaxing Environment: Set the tone for cooking by playing your favorite music, lighting candles, or opening a window to let in natural light and air. Creating a relaxing and pleasant ambiance can make cooking more enjoyable.

Prep in Advance: Take advantage of downtime during the week to prepare ingredients or even entire meals in advance. To make cooking easier and less stressful on busy weeknights, chop vegetables, marinade proteins, or pre-cook grains.

Cook Mindfully: While cooking, engage your senses and pay attention to the colors, textures, and scents of the food. Cooking thoughtfully can help reduce stress and increase enjoyment of the cooking process.

Don't be scared to get creative in the kitchen and try out new ingredients and dishes. Cooking is a form of self-expression, so have fun trying new flavors and techniques to make tasty and nutritious meals.

Cooking and sharing meals with loved ones may be a bonding experience that is both enjoyable and fulfilling. Invite friends and family to join you in the kitchen, or throw a potluck meal to enjoy wonderful cuisine and good company.

By adopting these suggestions and strategies into your cooking practice, you can make glaucoma-friendly meals enjoyable and stress-free, benefiting your entire health and well-being.

CHAPTER FIVE

Breakfast Recipes for Eye Health.

Introduction: Glaucoma is a collection of eye disorders that cause damage to the optic nerve, usually as a result of increased pressure inside the eye. While there is no treatment for glaucoma, certain lifestyle changes, such as dietary changes, can help manage the disease and lower the risk of progression. A well-balanced diet rich in nutrients needed for eye health, such as antioxidants, vitamins, and minerals, can help to improve general eye performance.

This cookbook attempts to provide delicious breakfast recipes that support eye health, with a focus on people who are concerned about or have glaucoma.

Quick and Nutritious Breakfast Ideas:

In today's hectic environment, many people struggle to find time for a healthy breakfast. However, beginning the day with a nutritious meal is critical, particularly for people with glaucoma. Quick breakfast selections should focus on nutrient density and convenience. Overnight oats, yogurt parfaits with fruits and nuts, and whole-grain toast topped with avocado and eggs are all great options. These meals are not only quick to prepare, but they also contain important nutrients such as fiber, vitamins, and healthy fats, which promote eye health and overall well-being.

Incorporating Fruits and Vegetables into Morning Meals: Fruits and vegetables are high in antioxidants such as vitamins A, C, and E, which help protect the eyes from oxidative damage and lower the risk of glaucoma progression. Breakfast is the optimum time to integrate these nutrient-dense foods into your diet. Green smoothies made with leafy greens, berries, and citrus fruits, as well as vegetable frittatas filled with colorful peppers, spinach, and tomatoes, are excellent choices. Individuals can ensure a varied range of nutrients necessary for keeping healthy eyes by consuming a variety of fruits and vegetables in their morning meals.

The Importance of Protein and Fibre for Maintained Energy: Protein and fiber are crucial nutrients that help regulate blood sugar levels and offer maintained energy throughout the day, making them critical components of a glaucoma prevention diet. Breakfast meals should include lean protein sources like eggs, Greek yogurt, or plant-based alternatives like tofu or lentils, as well as high-fiber foods like whole grains, nuts, seeds, and fruits. Incorporating these nutrients into breakfast can help people feel full, keep their energy levels up, and improve overall eye health by maintaining stable blood flow to the optic nerve.

Simple Smoothies and Muesli Recipes: Smoothies and muesli are versatile breakfast options that may be customized with a variety of eye-healthy ingredients. Smoothies can include leafy greens, antioxidant-rich fruits, nuts, seeds, and plant-based protein sources such as hemp or pea protein powder. Similarly, muesli can be flavored with fruits, nuts, seeds, and spices such as cinnamon, which contains anti-inflammatory qualities. These recipes provide a practical method to pack numerous nutrients into a single meal, making them great for people wishing to improve their breakfast for eye health while remaining simple and easy to prepare.

Finally, a nutritious breakfast is an essential component of a glaucoma-prevention diet. Individuals can support their eye health and overall well-being by including quick and healthy meal ideas, focusing on fruits and vegetables, emphasizing the importance of protein and fiber, and including simple smoothie and muesli dishes. Making these dietary modifications can help supplement other glaucoma control measures and lead to a better lifestyle in the long run.

Lunchtime Favourites: Nutritious Midday Meals

A well-balanced diet is essential for preserving eye health and preventing diseases like glaucoma.

The Lunchtime Favourites section of the Glaucoma Prevention Diet Cookbook contains a variety of delicious noon meal alternatives to keep you full and energized throughout the day. Let's go into the concepts mentioned in this section:

Salads are an excellent way to include a variety of nutrients in your diet while keeping it light and refreshing. To avoid glaucoma, it is critical to focus on substances high in antioxidants, vitamins, and minerals that promote eye health. Leafy greens like spinach, kale, and rocket are ideal choices since they include lutein and zeaxanthin, two antioxidants that have been shown to improve eye health by lowering the risk of age-related macular degeneration and other disorders.

Incorporating colorful vegetables such as bell peppers, carrots, and tomatoes into your salad also provides a plethora of vitamins A, C, and E, all of which play important roles in keeping healthy vision and guarding against oxidative stress. Consider adding lean protein sources like grilled chicken, chickpeas, or tofu. Nuts, seeds, and avocado are also excellent additions, providing healthy fats and extra nutrients.

Protein-Rich Lunch Options for Sustained Energy:

Protein is needed to form and repair tissues, including those in the eyes. Incorporating protein-rich foods into your lunch can help you stay energized throughout the afternoon while also improving your overall health. Choose lean foods such as grilled fish, chicken breast, turkey, or lentils and beans.

Combining protein with complex carbohydrates and healthy fats can boost satiety and energy levels. Consider a quinoa salad with black beans and avocado, or grilled fish wrapped in whole-grain tortillas and vegetables.

These alternatives provide a well-balanced nutritional profile that will keep you full and focused until your next meal.

Adding Whole Grains to Your Lunch Routine:

Whole grains are high in fiber, vitamins, and minerals, all of which benefit overall health, including eye health. They assist in managing blood sugar levels, improve digestion, and lower the risk of chronic diseases like diabetes and heart disease, both of which are linked to an increased risk of glaucoma.

Incorporating whole grains into your lunch routine is as simple as replacing refined grains with whole grain counterparts. Choose from brown rice, quinoa, barley, full-grain bread, and pasta. These solutions provide consistent energy release, keeping you full and pleased while promoting good health.

CHAPTER SIX

On hurried days, having portable lunch options at your disposal is critical for maintaining a balanced diet and avoiding glaucoma. Portable meals should be simple to pack, need little prep, and stay fresh for several hours.

Consider whole grain wraps with lean protein, vegetables, and hummus, or mason jar salads with substantial components like grains, beans, vegetables, and a tasty vinaigrette. Snack boxes including a variety of healthful ingredients, such as sliced fruits, vegetables, nuts, and cheese, are also convenient for on-the-go consumption.

By implementing these ideas into your lunchtime routine, you can prepare nutritional meals that promote eye health and overall well-being, perhaps lowering your risk of glaucoma and other eye diseases over time.

Delicious Dinners to Prevent Glaucoma

When it comes to managing glaucoma, food is just as important as medical treatment. A Glaucoma Prevention Diet Cookbook is a detailed guide to preparing delicious meals that not only satisfy your taste buds but also help to maintain eye health. Let's look at some of the important topics addressed in this cookbook, with a particular emphasis on dinners:

Flavorful and Nutritious Dinner Recipes: Dinner is frequently regarded as the primary meal of the day, and it provides an ideal opportunity to consume important nutrients while enjoying delicious foods. The Glaucoma Prevention Diet Cookbook includes a variety of delectable recipes that have been carefully created to give both nutritional value and palatability. From nourishing soups to tantalizing main dishes, these recipes are intended to make following a glaucoma-friendly diet a pleasurable experience.

Incorporating Lean Proteins and Healthy Fats: Proteins are essential for maintaining eye health since they serve as building blocks for various eye tissues. Lean proteins like skinless fowl, fish, tofu, and lentils are featured in the cookbook's evening meals. These protein sources are not just low in saturated fats, but also high in nutrients like omega-3 fatty acids, which have been associated with a lower risk of glaucoma progression. Furthermore, the cookbook emphasizes the use of healthy fats, such as those found in olive oil, avocado, and almonds, to promote overall eye health while also improving the flavor and texture of dishes.

Colorful vegetables are an important part of a glaucoma-preventive diet because they include a lot of antioxidants, which help fight oxidative stress and inflammation in the eyes.

The guidebook recommends combining a variety of colorful veggies into dinner preparations to maximize their eye-protective properties.

From leafy greens like kale and spinach to antioxidant-rich bell peppers and carrots, each recipe is designed to highlight the various flavors and textures of these healthful items. Individuals can nourish their eyes while eating a colorful array of vegetables for dinner.

One-Pot Meals for Easy Cleanup: Convenience is essential, especially when preparing dinner after a long day.

The Glaucoma Prevention Diet Cookbook includes a variety of one-pot recipes that simplify the cooking process and reduce cleanup.

These dishes are designed to be simple but savory, allowing people to prepare a nutritious dinner without spending hours in the kitchen. These recipes save time and effort by using only one pot or skillet, making it easier to stick to a healthy eating plan continuously.

Nutritious snack alternatives to satisfy hunger in between meals:

Snacking does not have to entail eating processed meals high in sugar and fat. Instead, go for nutrient-dense foods that will keep you feeling full and energized until your next meal. Here are a few nutritious snack ideas:

Snack on fresh fruits and vegetables, which are high in vitamins, minerals, and antioxidants while being low in calories. Choose carrot sticks, apple slices, or cherry tomatoes for a crunchy and refreshing snack.

Greek yogurt, high in protein and probiotics, is a nutritious snack that can help curb hunger. For extra flavor and nutrition, top with fresh berries or a sprinkle of nuts and seeds.

For prolonged energy, choose whole grain crackers or rice cakes, which include complex carbs. For a well-balanced snack, top with avocado, hummus, or lean protein such as turkey or chicken.

Top celery sticks with almond or peanut butter for a crisp and delicious snack high in healthy fats and protein. Just be aware of portion amounts to avoid overdoing the calories.

For a tasty and low-calorie snack, try air-popped popcorn seasoned with herbs or nutritional yeast instead of butter.

CHAPTER SEVEN

The importance of portion control during snacking:

While snacking can be a healthy habit, it's important to practice portion control to avoid consuming too many calories. Even healthful meals can cause weight gain if consumed in high quantities.

Use smaller plates or bowls to mislead your brain into thinking you're eating more, resulting in more satisfaction with fewer portions.

To avoid mindless munching, pre-portion foods into individual servings. This is especially useful for items that are easy to overeat, such as nuts and trail mix.

Assess hunger indicators before snacking to see if you're actually hungry or eating out of habit. Choose snacks that will satisfy your hunger without making you feel too full.

Be alert when eating: Avoid distractions like TV or phone use while munching. Instead, concentrate on the flavor, texture, and satisfaction of your food, which might help you avoid overeating.

Incorporating nuts and seeds to improve eye health:

Nuts and seeds are nutritious powerhouses that provide numerous health advantages, including improved eye health. They are high in antioxidants, vitamins, and minerals, which can help prevent age-related eye disorders such as glaucoma. Here's how to include nuts and seeds in your diet for better eye health:

Snack on a variety of nuts and seeds to get different nutrients. For example, almonds are strong in vitamin E, which has been associated with a lower risk of cataracts, and flaxseeds are high in omega-3 fatty acids, which may help prevent dry eye syndrome.

Make your own trail mix by combining nuts and seeds like almonds, walnuts, pumpkin seeds, and sunflower seeds. This not only delivers a variety of nutrients but also enhances the flavor and texture of your food.

Spread nut butter like almond, peanut, or cashew on whole grain crackers or apple slices for a healthful snack. Nut butters are an easy way to incorporate the nutritional advantages of nuts into your diet while also adding protein and healthy fats.

Add chia, flaxseed, or hemp seeds to salads, yogurt, or smoothies for a nutritional boost. Seeds are adaptable and can be added to several foods to improve both flavor and nutritional content.

Homemade snack recipes for easy on-the-go eating:

Making your own snacks at home allows you to manage the ingredients and customize the flavors to your liking. Here are some homemade snack ideas ideal for on-the-go convenience:

Energy balls are bite-sized treats made with oats, nut butter, and honey, with added dried fruit, nuts, and seeds. They're simple to prepare ahead of time and consume when you need a quick energy boost.

Serve fresh veggies (e.g. carrots, cucumbers, bell peppers) with homemade yogurt dip flavored with herbs and spices. This snack contains fiber, vitamins, and probiotics, all of which promote intestinal health.

Make baked kale chips by tossing kale leaves with olive oil, salt, and seasonings. Bake until crispy for a healthy snack alternative to potato chips. Kale is high in lutein and zeaxanthin, antioxidants that may help prevent macular degeneration.

Make homemade granola bars with rolled oats, nuts, seeds, dried fruit, and a binder such as honey or maple syrup. These bars are ideal for filling hunger on the go and may be customized with your preferred ingredients.

By adopting these concepts into your snacking routine and experimenting with homemade snack recipes, you may improve your general health and help avoid glaucoma with a nutritious diet. Remember to eat your snacks consciously and in moderation, paying attention to portion sizes and hunger cues for the best health results.

Desserts and Treats: Indulge without Compromise

When it comes to living a healthy lifestyle, desserts are frequently viewed as an indulgence to be avoided. However, with the appropriate technique, you may indulge in tasty delights without jeopardizing your health goals. A Glaucoma Prevention Diet Cookbook understands the need for balance and provides a choice of dessert options that not only satisfy your sweet appetite but also promote overall health.

One of the guiding concepts of a Glaucoma Prevention Diet Cookbook is to offer nutritious and appealing options. Instead of using refined sugars and processed ingredients, these recipes focus on natural sweeteners like honey, maple syrup, and fruit purees. Desserts can be made more flavorful and nutritious by using whole ingredients.

Instead of classic brownies made with refined flour and sugar, you may look up recipes for black bean brownies sweetened with dates or banana bread prepared with almond flour and no additional sugars. These alternatives not only fulfill sweet cravings, but they also provide important nutrients like fiber, antioxidants, and healthy fats.

Importance of moderation in dessert consumption.

While it is vital to consume sweets in proportion, it is equally critical to recognize that moderation means various things to different people. Some people love a tiny treat every day, while others only eat dessert on exceptional occasions.

By paying attention to how particular foods make you feel, you may make better decisions about when and how much dessert to have.

The cookbook also includes portion control tips, such as using smaller plates, savoring each bite, and sharing sweets with others. Dessert can be part of a balanced diet without making you feel guilty or jeopardizing your health if you practice moderation and mindful eating.

Adding fruits to dessert recipes

Fruits are naturally delicious, but they also include vitamins, minerals, and antioxidants that promote eye health and overall well-being. A Glaucoma Prevention Diet Cookbook recommends using fresh or frozen fruits in dessert recipes to give sweetness and flavor without the need for additional sugars.

For example, you may find recipes for fruit crisps made with apples, berries, and peaches, as well as fruit sorbets sweetened with ripe bananas or mangoes. Incorporating a variety of fruits into your desserts allows you to experience a diversity of flavors and textures while enjoying the nutritional advantages of these healthy components.

Dessert alternatives with minimal sugar and carbohydrate content

A Glaucoma Prevention Diet Cookbook provides a variety of solutions to fulfill sweet desires without creating blood sugar rises. These recipes frequently use alternative sweeteners like stevia, erythritol, or monk fruit extract to deliver sweetness without the added calories or carbohydrates found in typical sweets.

Low-carb desserts may also contain ingredients like almond flour, coconut flour, or flaxseed meal, which lower carbohydrate content while adding fiber and beneficial fats. From sugar-free cheesecakes to keto-friendly cookies, there are lots of decadent treats to suit your dietary preferences and health objectives.

Finally, a Glaucoma Prevention Diet Cookbook recognizes that desserts can be part of a healthy diet and provides a choice of options to please your sweet craving while supporting overall health and wellness. You may enjoy tasty sweets without compromising your nutritional objectives or jeopardizing your eye health if you focus on full ingredients, moderation, and mindful eating.

The Glaucoma Prevention Diet Cookbook must include recipes high in nutrients that promote eye health, particularly antioxidants, vitamins, minerals, and omega-3 fatty acids. Here are several recipes suited for people wishing to avoid or manage glaucoma:

Salmon Salad with Leafy Greens: This refreshing salad contains omega-3 fatty acids from salmon as well as antioxidants from leafy greens such as spinach and kale.

Quinoa and Vegetable Stir-Fry: This colorful stir-fry combines quinoa, a whole grain high in protein and fiber, with a variety of vegetables such as bell peppers, broccoli, and carrots, which provide a variety of vitamins and minerals.

Berry Smoothie with Flaxseeds: A tasty smoothie made with antioxidant-rich berries (blueberries, strawberries, or raspberries) and flaxseeds, which are strong in omega-3 fatty acids and fiber.

Roasted Brussels Sprouts with Almonds: Brussels sprouts are high in vitamins C and K, both of which are beneficial to eye health. Roasting them with almonds provides a crispy texture and additional nutrients.

Grilled Chicken with Garlic and Herbs: Combining lean chicken protein with garlic and herbs improves flavor while also providing antioxidant and anti-inflammatory effects.

Spinach & Feta Stuffed Bell Peppers: Bell peppers are high in vitamin C and beta-carotene, which can help prevent eye problems. Stuffing them with spinach and feta cheese results in a delicious and nutritious meal.

Tuna Salad Lettuce Wraps: Tuna contains omega-3 fatty acids, and lettuce leaves give moisture and fiber. Adding colorful veggies, such as tomatoes and cucumbers, improves the nutritious profile.

Sweet Potato and Kale Hash: Sweet potatoes include beta-carotene, which is turned into vitamin A in the body and is necessary for eye health. Kale adds vitamins and nutrients to this hearty stew.

: Walnuts are high in omega-3 fatty acids and antioxidants, while cranberries give a sweet and tangy flavor as well as more antioxidants. When combined with quinoa, this salad creates a healthful and filling dinner.

Baked Cod with Lemon and Herbs: Cod is a lean protein source containing omega-3 fatty acids. Baking with lemon and herbs adds flavor while keeping the dish light and healthful.

30-days meal plan for patients who want to prevent glaucoma:

Day 1:

Breakfast: Berry smoothie with flaxseed.

Snack: Carrot Sticks and Hummus.

Lunch: Quinoa and vegetable stir-fry.

Snack: Greek Yoghurt and Berries.

Dinner: Grilled chicken with garlic and herbs, served with roasted Brussels sprouts and almonds.

Day 2:

Breakfast: Spinach and Mushroom Omelette.

Snack: Apple slices and almond butter.

Lunch: Salmon salad with leafy greens.

Snack: Walnut and Cranberry Quinoa Salad.

Dinner: Sweet potato and kale hash.

Continue this routine, making sure to eat a variety of nutrient-dense meals every day, such as fruits, vegetables, lean meats, whole grains, and healthy fats. Adjust portion sizes to meet individual calorie demands and tastes, and stay hydrated with water throughout the day. Also, advise people to check with their healthcare physician or a trained dietitian for personalized dietary advice.

In conclusion, the Glaucoma Prevention Diet Cookbook contains a treasure trove of dinner recipes designed to promote eye health while tantalizing your taste buds. Individuals can enjoy tasty dinners that contribute to their general well-being and help prevent glaucoma progression by incorporating lean proteins, healthy fats, colorful veggies, and one-pot meal alternatives.

Snack Attack: Healthy Options for Any Time of Day!

Snacking can be a hindrance to sticking to a balanced diet. However, with the correct strategy and choices, snacking can help you achieve your overall health goals, including eye health in the case of glaucoma prevention.

THE END

www.ingramcontent.com/pod-product-compliance
Lightning Source LLC
Chambersburg PA
CBHW061304250726
48653CB00002B/766